Pregnancy Guide For First Time Moms:

Month By Month Guidance For a Healthy Pregnancy

By

Eva Delano

Table of Contents

Introduction 5

Chapter 1. How to Prepare Yourself For Pregnancy 7

Chapter 2. What You Should Eat While You Are Pregnant . 16

Chapter 3. What You Must Not Eat 19

Chapter 4. Medications Allowed For You 21

Chapter 5. Medications You Cannot Take During Pregnancy 23

Chapter 6. Travelling Tips For Pregnant Women 24

Chapter 7. Prenatal Checkups 26

Chapter 8. Body Changes to Expect During Pregnancy 28

Chapter 9. Emotional Changes 30

Conclusion 32

Thank You Page 33

Pregnancy Guide For First Time Moms: Month By Month Guidance For a Healthy Pregnancy

By Eva Delano

© Copyright 2015 Eva Delano

Reproduction or translation of any part of this work beyond that permitted by section 107 or 108 of the 1976 United States Copyright Act without permission of the copyright owner is unlawful. Requests for permission or further information should be addressed to the author.

This publication is designed to provide accurate and authoritative information in regard to the subject matter covered. This work is sold with the understanding that the publisher is not engaged in rendering legal, accounting, or other professional services. If legal advice or other expert assistance is required, the services of a competent professional person should be sought.

First Published, 2015

Printed in the United States of America

Introduction

Even if the child is only carried by the woman, it does not mean that the journey of pregnancy should only be taken by the woman. As a couple, both of you are responsible for the child that will soon see the world. For you to make the child healthy and happy as soon as he or she is born, there things that you need to do as a mother to prepare the child especially when it comes to their health and your partner should be involved in it too.

From the day that you find out that you are pregnant until the baby is born, you are responsible for the child's health, but the most important thing is to keep yourself healthy and eat the right kinds of food to nourish your child. It's a reality that women don't know everything yet about pregnancy yet which is why this book was written for you because no one is an expert especially if it's their first time to be a mom. You will find here what you need to eat so that your baby will get the proper nutrients and also to keep you strong enough to go through the whole pregnancy. In case you need to take any medication, you will read here what are safe for you to take and what aren't.

You will also know proper exercises so that you can still stay fit even if you are pregnant and if you like to travel, you will be given some tips on how travel even if you are pregnant. Each stage of pregnancy will also be described here because the body goes through certain changes during pregnancy and it's important that you know what these changes are. Some women go through potential issues before the baby and in case you have these issues, you will know more about them from this book.

Pregnancy is a beautiful journey that every woman deserves to take and when you see your child smiling at you, all of the hardships that you have gone through while you were pregnant will suddenly go away so there's nothing to be afraid of because you are lucky enough to be given a child to take care of. After you have finished reading this book, you will become more ready and your pregnancy fears will go away.

Chapter 1. How to Prepare Yourself For Pregnancy

Before anything else, you need to talk to your partner about pregnancy and when will they be ready to go through it with you. You need discuss as a couple what will be the parenting issues, what you will expect, how it will change your priorities, and especially when especially parenting techniques. The younger years when growing up are the most crucial because it will help shape them as a person and they are still very fragile to the world they see. You also need to find out how your finances will go as couple and how you will fix your funds in order to sustain the pregnancy and the baby. If you are taking pregnancy prevention pills, you need to stop taking it for a few months before you are planning to get pregnant because even if your cycle used to be every 27 or 32 days, it will not be like how it was before after you have taken the birth control pills. Your hormone levels will take a little time to get back to its normal state again so you need to get rid of the pills and you will also know when you are ovulating with your new cycle.

You need to say goodbye to partying for a while because both alcohol and smoking are really bad for pregnancy. If you are a heavy smoker, you need to stop a few months before you are planning to get pregnant because it can affect your fertility and as for him, it could cause his sperm count to become lower so you both need to stop partying because even if you are just a secondhand smoker, it could still affect you. Smoking cigarettes and drinking alcohol could lead to miscarriage, birth defects, and other problems. So if you don't want to deal with a lot of complications after your child is born, you need to stop partying. You also cannot just stop smoking only if you find out that you are pregnant because this could give your system a shock. Caffeine is a regular part of anyone's day, but if you will conceive, you need to lower down your intake and you can no longer take 4 cups of coffee in a day because too much caffeine can be a factor to miscarriage. This does not only mean lessen your coffee intake, but all other sources of caffeine as well.

You also need to monitor your weight whether you are overweight or underweight because 10 to 15 pounds heavier than your ideal weight could affect pregnancy and if you are way below the ideal weight, you need to gain a few extra pounds. Always find out the pounds that you need to lose or gain because if you do not have a BMI that falls between 19 and 24, you need to do something about your weight. For any couple who wants to start a family life, planning on where your funds are bound to go is one of the most important things because you know you will need money for giving birth, diapers, baby stuff, education plans, and all the other things that involve raising a kid. Even if you have a lot of extra cash, that is totally fine because it is better to have excess rather than being short on funds.

There might also some extra expenses that might come during your pregnancy so it is better to be prepared for that. Prenatal supplements especially folic acid will help if you start taking it 3 to 6 months before you want to get pregnant will help a lot. Supplements could supply you with at least 400 milligrams of folic acid in a day and if you take this, it could help lessen by 70% the chances of developing brain and spine defects for your baby. Multivitamins will have the sufficient amount of nutrients that you and your baby will need during the 9 months. Multivitamins also has iron that will prevent anemia and also calcium for stronger bones and teeth. Starting this habit early will help you get it into your routine even after you have given birth. They say that sleep is important especially while you are growing up, but sleep is important no matter what stage of life you are in.

Before getting pregnant, you need to get lots of sleep because when the baby is there, you will be deprived of sleep when your baby will wake you up in the middle of the night. While you are pregnant, you will also have a hard time getting enough sleep because you can experience heartburn occasionally and you will have to pee more often in the middle of the night. Getting enough sleep can also help your chances of becoming pregnant because lack of sleep can also affect your ovulation. If you are stressed a lot, this will get in the way of you becoming pregnant because it can get in the way of your ovulation and the embryo might not be able to implant itself into the uterine walls. Those who are type-A personality born tend to get even more stressed while they are pregnant so you need to check on your emotional state now.

You should be calm enough to go through this next chapter of your life and you need to find out what you can do to lessen your stress level. You can try going out for a run, contacting people you trust, or writing down some thoughts anytime something is bothering you can help lessen your stress level. Before the baby comes, you can spend ample time with your partner. Take pictures of your pregnancy journey because once the baby is born, the luxury of time will be lessen and these pictures you have taken will help keep you smiling. When your child gets old enough to appreciate photos, they will love seeing the pictures you have taken while they were still inside your womb and this could be a fun time for them to ask you things about how they were while still inside your womb. This will remind your child how happy you are as a couple before and after they are born. If you are a couple who loves to dine out and find leisure in eating, you need to make a list of the places you want to try before getting pregnant because while you are pregnant, you will have morning sickness and occasional cravings. Even your palate is affected. You also won't be able to splurge on food like you used to when you already have a child because your meals will change a little bit and even the places you want to go to.

Living spaces can also be important when planning your pregnancy and thinking about the space you have now because you're going to need a little more space once you have a child. If you think that you need to move before getting pregnant, do it because you don't want to have all the stress and trouble of moving while you are pregnant especially when you are already 8 months pregnant. Doing it early will help you emotionally and you will be able to plan on other things once you have moved. This will trigger you to collaborate about your new living costs, but if you have enough living space, you don't have to move. If all of you will be comfortable, then you have nothing to worry about. If your job is demanding too much of your time, you might want to consider another job because you will need to spend more hours at home with your child and the stress that your job is giving you could affect your pregnancy.

Also make an observation of the new parents in your company if they are happy with their job. These are what must be pondered upon and talk to your boss if he or she can change your schedule or lessen your workload, but if your boss says that it can't be done, leave. You and your child are more important and there are other job opportunities out there that can give you better treatment. Try doing history check-up of your family about certain problems that might have caused them to take longer than usual to get pregnant. Low quality of eggs and blocked fallopian tubes cannot be acquired through heredity, but ovarian cysts and fibroids can be caused by your family's heredity. You can talk to your sister, cousin, mom, and aunts about their pregnancy journey and how long it took them to get pregnant, but that does not mean you will have the same. It's just good to inform them about your steps and they can also give you advice about being pregnant and some baby tips. 3 months before you get pregnant, you need to see your doctor and get results if you have chronic illnesses that you are not aware of like asthma, diabetes, heart illnesses, and malfunctioning thyroid glands. Your partner should also have himself checked to see that he has enough sperm count and he is healthy enough to produce a baby with you. The doctor could also ask you to do genetic testing to see if you have anything that can be detrimental to your health while you are pregnant and also what diseases are in the history of your genes. You need to make sure that you will be taking medications that will be safe for you and will not give any bad side effects.

You should also be at peace with your doctor and evaluate if you will be able to talk to them easily even after you have given birth because having a good relationship with your doctor is important. It is hard to seek advice from someone you are not comfortable with even if she is your doctor. Your doctor needs to give you the right answers to your questions every time and they should be very accommodating to all of your needs. Another person you need to visit is your dentist because oral health is connected with pregnancy and women who don't have healthy gums have a higher chance of experiencing a miscarriage, preeclampsia, and pre-term birth. Maintaining your teeth well can lessen the risk of miscarriage by 70%. If your hair is always colored, you might want to go back to your original hair color because doctors recommend that you need to decrease your exposure to chemicals while you are pregnant especially at the first trimester of your pregnancy because this is the time when the major organs of your baby are starting to develop. Ask your hairdresser what chemicals are in the hair color that they use or it is much better if you go back to your original hair color. It's also hard to maintain artificial hair color while you are pregnant.

Chapter 2. What You Should Eat While You Are Pregnant

Eggs – They only contain 90 calories and you get up to 12 vitamins and minerals by just eating on a day. Eggs are very packed with protein and each cell is made up of protein and this is how it will promote the growth and cell formation of your baby. There are eggs that also contain omega-3 fats that are important for vision and the development of the brain. The eggs that are DHA-enriched have the highest amount of omega-3s. Egg contains a lot of cholesterol, but very low saturated fat and studies show that it's the saturated fat that can damage your system not the cholesterol found in food. If your blood cholesterol is in top shape, you are safe to consume 1 to 2 eggs per day.

Salmon – Another great source of protein and omega-3 fats that are important for the brain development of your baby. It can also help with your mood and it does not contain a lot of mercury unlike mackerel, shark, and tilefish. Mercury is harmful to the development system of your baby.

Beans – Beans have a lot of variety and among all of the vegetables, they have the biggest amount of protein and fiber. Protein is important for your pregnancy, but so is fiber because when the function of the gastrointestinal tract becomes slower during pregnancy you can have a risk of being constipated and having hemorrhoids. Fiber will help with relieving and preventing them from happening. Fiber-rich foods have a ton of nutrients and this is why beans also contain folate, zinc, calcium, and of course iron.

Fruits and vegetables – By eating different varieties of fruits and vegetables, you are positive that you are getting the right nutrients that you and your baby both need. The different groups of fruits and vegetables have vitamins and minerals that are important. If you eat fruits and vegetables in the last stages of your pregnancy, the amniotic fluid helps the baby taste the food that you are eating so this is also a way for you to introduce your baby early to eating fruits and vegetables later on.

Lean meats – When you are buying meat, it should be at least 95% fat free especially beef and pork meat because they have choline. You need to avoid eating hotdogs and deli meats that are raw because you can have the risk of having bacteria and parasites like toxoplasma, listeria, and salmonella. You will pass this on to your baby.

Walnuts – This is a very rich source of omega-3 that is gotten from plants. Even if very little amount of DHA is provided by plant-based omega-3 fats, a ton of fiber and protein is available from walnuts.

Sweet potatoes – They are orange because of carotenoids and they later on get converted by our bodies to vitamin A. Even if too much consumption of vitamin A that is preformed can be a danger to your body, the carotenoids are only converted by the body to vitamin A if it is needed which means that vitamin A found in fruits and vegetables are okay to consume frequently. Sweet potatoes can also give you a good amount of vitamin C, fiber and of course folate.

Chapter 3. What You Must Not Eat

Undercooked foods – Unpasteurized eggs, rare meat, cookie dough, sushi, and eggnog may have parasites, viruses, and bacterial growth. To be safe from getting illnesses that are foodborne, check if the food is well-done by getting a food thermometer and the egg should not be runny.

Unpasteurized dairy, hot dogs, and luncheon meats – These types of food are susceptible to listeria monocytogenes. A kind of Bacteria that can lead to listeriosis, causes stillbirth, miscarriage, and serious health complications. Other foods that are processed like meat spreads, canned fish, and other seafood can also contain listeria. You can eat refrigerated seafood that is smoked when you eat it with a dish that is well-cooked. The luncheon meats and frankfurters are safe to eat as long as you 'cook' them. Fluids packages of hotdogs should not be spread to other utensils and where they are preparing food because it can still be a risk for having listeria. Always wash your hands after handling hotdog or other processed foods. Dairy foods that are unpasteurized should also be avoided because listeria could also be contaminating them.

Some seafood and fish - Avoid eating fish that have a lot of mercury content. These fishes are tilefish, king mackerel, and swordfish because their mercury content is higher than most of the fish that can be eaten. FDA said that pregnant women are allowed to eat 12 ounces of fishes that are low in mercury every week. Farmed and wild salmon, Pollock, tuna in the can, sardines, catfish and shrimp are other seafood that does not have a lot of mercury in them. Higher mercury content is found in Albacore tuna in comparison to the canned light tuna and pregnant women should only consume 6 ounces of this in a week.

Vegetables sprouts that are raw – This is very dangerous because it is hard to wash out the bacteria that are present in them and the FDA advises not to eat them at all regardless of pregnancy. Sprouts that are cooked well causes no harm to health

Chapter 4. Medications Allowed For You

For pain relief – You can always try a cold compress for your headache or muscle pain if that does not do the trick, your doctor might tell you to take acetaminophen which is an active component in Tylenol. It is safe to consume this drug, but you have to keep yourself from taking nonsteroidal anti-inflammatory medication like ibuprofen, and naproxen. Another medication to be avoided is aspirin and if you drink them on the early stages of pregnancy and also before giving birth can lead to birth defects and miscarriage.

For colds and allergies – For you to be able to avoid getting cough and colds, you can try drinking a lot of warm liquids and saline nasal spray can take away stuffiness. Even if you have cough and colds while you are pregnant, you should not be worried. Consider getting flu shots but they get more serious during pregnancy and can later on lead to respiratory complications. If allergies and colds give you difficulty with sleeping, your doctor can tell you to take antihistamine chlorpheniramine which is very safe for you as long as you are no longer in your first trimester because it does not cause birth defects.

Digestive discomfort – This can cause constipation, heartburn, and hemorrhoids. Your doctor will recommend you to take antacid if natural remedies are not effective for you. In case the antacid is not enough to eliminate discomfort, the next thing that your Doctor will ask you to take is Carafate which is a drug that protects the lining of the stomach and coats it. To prevent digestive discomfort, you can eat foods that are rich in fiber and drink lots of water.

Chapter 5. Medications You Cannot Take During Pregnancy

Pain relievers – Naproxen, ibuprofen, and aspirin must never be taken during pregnancy.

Gastrointestinal problems – This is common during pregnancy and this happens when the body slows down on digestion to absorb all of the nutrients found in food. This could be the cause of constipation, bloating, heartburn, and irregular bowel movements. Do not take Pepto-Bismol and Kaopectate.

For colds – Having colds while you are pregnant can be very uncomfortable but taking over the counter drugs are not recommended because they have brompheniramine, pseudoephredrine, and chlorpheniramine. Before buying the medication, ask your doctor which you can take that does not contain these 3 components.

Chapter 6. Travelling Tips For Pregnant Women

Be wise with your destination

Avoid choosing places where it will take long hours of flight because it will be very uncomfortable for you. Choose places that will only 2 to 3 hours for you to get there and no long airport transfers.

Plan early

Make an itinerary and write down the things that you will need to take with you so you will not forget them.

Pack what you need

If you will be walking a lot during your travel, take trainers or comfortable shoes with you. Blister pads are also a must to wear with your shoes even if they are comfortable. Always pack flat shoes for short distance walks.

Take breaks if you need to

You don't have to be walking all the time and walking while being pregnant can be a little more tiring than when you are not pregnant. Sleep if you have to and it will allow you to recharge so you can enjoy more.

Common sense

Avoid the activities that will give you a risk of falling like skydiving, rock climbing, and other difficult sports.

Chapter 7. Prenatal Checkups

Your doctor will first discuss with you about the state of your health and your doctor will have questions that she wants you to answer honestly. You will be asked the following questions:

- The date of your last menstrual period.

- If you have problems with your health like STDs, high blood pressure, or diabetes.

- If you've gotten pregnant before, but was not successful.

- If you are taking any medications or if you are allergic to any.

- How your lifestyle is - if you smoke and drink alcohol.

- If you exercise regularly.

- What kind of stress you have.

- Safety of your living environment.

- The health history of your family.

- The health history of your partner.

They will also check on your weight, your blood pressure, and they will do a physical and pelvic exam. Your urine will be tested if you have any infection, check your blood for anemia, HIV, but if you say no, they will not do a test on that. A pap smear will also be done to you to check for cervical cancer and you will also be told to take 600 mg of folic acid daily.

Chapter 8. Body Changes to Expect During Pregnancy

First 6 to 14 weeks

You will experience nausea which happens early during the day, but could last the entire day. You will also notice your breasts starting to sore and grow. The areolas will also grow bigger and become darker. Another change that is you will start to feel fatigued and have body aches because of the hormones during the first stages.

Next 14 to 22 weeks

Your abdomen will start to grow bigger and this is the most obvious physical change you will see. Your weight will increase by a few pounds or more and you will start to develop stretch marks which usually last for a long time even after pregnancy. You can gain up to 10 to 15 pounds if you do not watch what you eat and ideally you should only consume 300 more calories than your usual caloric intake.

Next 23 to 36 weeks

Your digestive system will start to slow down and the bigger uterine size will put more pressure on the intestinal tract which could be a risk for vomiting, hemorrhoids, and nausea. To prevent this, you should always take prenatal vitamins for your nutrients and taking folic acid during the early stages of pregnancy will help prevent this.

Chapter 9. Emotional Changes

You will be moody and you will have heightened emotions. Hormonal changes during pregnancy trigger mood swings. When you are adapting to a new chapter of life after the baby has been born, you can feel sad and some women go through post-partum depression. Don't hesitate to seek help if you need to.

First trimester

Not a lot of changes in the emotions can be experienced during this stage, but women will still feel anxious during this time because they think that they could still lose their baby which is a normal feeling.

Second trimester

When the anxiety stage is done which happens in the first trimester, there are emotional changes that will start to happen during the second trimester. Women will start to become more conscious about their body because of the weight they are gaining and this could cause them to have a low self-esteem.

Third trimester

As soon as the third trimester enters, women are waiting for child birth and they are excited about becoming a mom. They no longer fear that they will lose the baby, but a new kind of anxiety will happen - they will worry about the arrival of the baby. Women will also have fears about labor and birth which commonly happens when they are already on their last stages of pregnancy.

Conclusion

These are the things you will need to go through and consider during pregnancy because you have another life inside of you. It is a beautiful journey and you need to make all of the necessary preparations so you can give birth to a healthy and happy baby.

Thank You Page

I want to personally thank you for reading my book. I hope you found information in this book useful and I would be very grateful if you could leave your honest review about this book. I certainly want to thank you in advance for doing this.

If you have the time, you can check my other books too.

www.ingramcontent.com/pod-product-compliance
Lightning Source LLC
LaVergne TN
LVHW021745060526
838200LV00052B/3487